Cyclic Vomiting Syndrome

Tests, Causes and Treatment Options

John Smith MA

Editor in Chief: *M Awad MD*

© 2011 Andale Publishing, LLC

All Rights Reserved worldwide under the Berne Convention. May not be copied or distributed without prior written permission by the publisher. If you have this book or an electronic document and didn't pay for it, then the author didn't get a fair share. Please consider paying for your copy. Thank you!

Printed in the United States of America

ISBN: **978-1467925198**

Contents

One: What is Cyclic Vomiting Syndrome (CVS)? 5

Two: Why do you get CVS? 11

Three: Common symptoms and signs of CVS 19

Four: Diagnosis 27

Five: Treatment 55

    Alternative Therapies 61

Six: Internet Resources/Further Reading 79

Seven: Glossary of Medical Terms 93

Eight: References 113

One: What is Cyclic Vomiting Syndrome (CVS)?

Cyclic Vomiting Syndrome (CVS) is a condition in which a person suffers from severe attacks of nausea and vomiting. CVS was first noted by Samuel Gee in 1982. Although a long time has passed, doctors are still unable to determine what causes CVS. Adults and children are equally vulnerable to this condition -- which is periodic. One day you may be perfectly normal and healthy. And the very next day, you may be vomiting. Then again, the next day you may be healthy and after a day or two or few days, you may again suffer from an episode of vomiting. This is why this condition is called recurrent. However, when the condition persists for a long time, you may start suffering from nausea during the normal periods too.

Each period of vomiting usually lasts for a minimum of 24 hours. The first hour is the hardest with extreme nausea and excessive vomiting. But then after 4 to 8 hours, the severity of the condition begins to decline. Every episode usually starts early in the morning, at about 2 - 4 am or at the time when you wake up. After the episode ends and vomits stop, you may be back to normal within 5 hours. When the condition is at its worst, you may experience up to 25 vomits per day.

Although vomiting is the most prominent symptom when you suffer from CVS, you may have other symptoms such as abdominal pain, diarrhea, headaches, or fever. According to most patients, the most distressing symptom when suffering from CVS is nausea. In CVS, you experience nausea all the time during a CVS attack and it can become very annoying and disturbing. Without treatment, the only time when you get rid of this feeling is when you are asleep or the episode is over.

CVS is a common condition among children. According to a number of studies, 2.3 percent children in Western Australia, 1.9 percent school-going children in Aberdeen, Scotland, and 4 out of every 100,000 children in Ireland may have CVS.

If you are suffering from CVS, this means that you will be sick about 10 percent of the time while the condition lasts, which could be months or years. This can make this condition a disabler, leaving you unable to take part in different activities due to the feeling of sickness or nausea that it causes. Also, more than half of CVS patients need IV fluids to be supplied to their bodies because vomiting can lead to dehydration. According to estimates, the average CVS patient suffers about $17000 financially when you suffer from CVS. This includes treatments costs, testing expenses and the financial loss you may suffer due to being absent from work.

If you are an adult, CVS can cause a lot of problems for you. You may ignore it at first and try to take it lightly which can lead to a wrong diagnosis of the condition, as happens in many cases. A wrong diagnosis will make the symptoms even worse and make your body weaker. It will also greatly hamper your work-routine and you may feel unable to work on many days when the vomiting episodes occur. A number of studies show that if you are an adult, you are at a high risk of getting an incorrect CVS diagnosis. Therefore, a proper knowledge of the symptoms of CVS is very important.

Although CVS affects people from all race and ethnicities, Caucasians are more often affected by it. The condition is slightly more likely to occur in women than men. The average age of children who suffer from CVS is about 4.8 years. But it can occur in infants as young as 6 days. In adults, although the average age of acquiring CVS is 21 years, the condition can occur as late as 78 years old.

There are four phases of CVS:

- **Prodrome.** This phase is the time when you feel that an episode of nausea and vomiting is about to begin. Usually, the most common symptom that you get is an abdominal pain which may last from few minutes to few hours. Taking a medication as soon as prodrome starts may stop an episode from occurring. But that's not always the case. Also, sometimes the episode is so sudden that you don't have time to take any medication before it starts. For instance, you may wake up one morning and immediately start vomiting without any forewarning.

- **Episode.** The episode may last up for a minimum of 24 hours. It is worst in the first hour when the feeling of nausea is strongest and you vomit a lot. It decreases in its severity gradually. You may find yourself unable to eat or drink while the episode lasts. Other prominent symptoms that you may experience during a CVS episode are pallor of skin, lethargy and a feeling of tiredness.

- **Recovery.** Once the nausea and vomiting ends, the recovery begins. From the start of an episode, it may take you up to 24 hours to completely be rid of symptoms like nausea. And then another 5 hours to return to normal so that you are able to eat and drink. The signs of the recovery phase are return of normal color to skin, return of appetite and end of lethargy.

- **Healthy interval/symptom-free interval**. This is the time between two episodes of CVS when you experience no CVS symptoms and your health appears normal.

Two: Why do you get CVS?

The exact cause of CVS is unknown. But doctors do have some hints at what can be the probable causes.

Migraine:

According to some recent studies if you suffer from migraine or if you have relatives who suffer from migraine, there is a high chance that you may also suffer from CVS. The studies show that people who have migraine in the family more often suffer from CVS than those who don't. About 82% of CVS patients have relatives who have migraine.

Genetic causes:

A genetic trait is something that you inherit from your parents. It's in your genes because either of your parents or both of them had it. Some studies show that your genetics are responsible for your CVS. A study shows that about 86 percent of CVS patients who are children have mothers who suffer from migraine. So the migraine of the mothers may have a link with CVS in the children. Doctors say that if a mother suffers from migraines, her children may have genetic mutations -- mutations that can result in a number of health problems. For example, in one case, a child who was suffering from CVS had a large piece of DNA missing. DNA is what contains your entire genetic information. It is a double-stranded structure which loops together. These two strands are separate and are held together by a third strand. Studies show that many children who suffer from CVS have a mutation in this third strand which is also called the D-loop. Another different feature in the DNA of CVS patients is that their DNA contains two elements 16519T and 3010A. These elements are not very frequently found in healthy people but are often in the DNA of CVS patients. The 16519T element was found to be six times more often in CVS patients who are children as compared to normal population. But these genetic factors which may possibly be responsible for CVS children are not the same for adults. In adults, these factors don't play any role in causing CVS.

Body response system:

When you are stressed and feel a lot of anxiety, your body reacts to this. The system in your body which is responsible for producing this reaction is called sympathetic system. The symptoms of the reaction produced by this system are pale skin, diarrhea, fever, tiredness and salivation. If you suffer from CVS, you experience similar symptoms. This had led the doctors to think that CVS is actually a result of some abnormality in the functioning of the sympathetic system. Doctors think that when the sympathetic system functions normally, it produces the symptoms mentioned above only when you are stressed. But when this system malfunctions, it starts producing the same symptoms suddenly, without any stress or anxiety. And that leads to CVS. A number of studies have shown such a link but it hasn't been proved yet.

An outcome of stress:

Doctors also believe that CVS may be an outcome of stress. Although your physical health may be perfectly alright, you may be depressed psychologically due to something that annoys you. This can lead to a reaction from the sympathetic system and can cause CVS. Often, the stomach starts malfunctioning due to the body's reaction to stress and this can induce nausea and lead to vomiting.

Triggers:

Although the causes of CVS are unknown, there are certain factors that increase the chances of a CVS attack. These are known as triggers and they vary from one person to another. Listed below are some triggers which are quite common among CVS patients:

- **Infection.** This is the most common trigger. An infection of the gastrointestinal tract can lead to an upset stomach or vomiting. And that can immediately trigger a CVS episode.

- **Excitement.** There are two types of excitement – one that is positive and the other that is negative. For example, if you are excited about something and it is worrying you a lot and stressing you, it is a negative type of excitement. But if you are happily excited about something, for instance a birthday party or a trip, that is a positive kind of excitement. Studies show that both of these types of excitement can trigger a CVS episode. If you are positively excited, the chances of a CVS episode are even higher than when you are negatively excited!

- **Cold and Flu.** Infections such as when you catch a cold or get flu can also trigger CVS attacks.

- **Foods.** This is a very common trigger factor. Sometimes, certain people can trigger their CVS episodes simply by eating certain foods. You may not be allergic to some food but your CVS may be sensitive to that food. For instance, you may be a chocolate lover and you may have been eating chocolate without any problems. But if your CVS is sensitive to chocolate, you may trigger a CVS attack as soon as you eat a chocolate. This goes the same for a number of foods such as cheese or milk. Every person's CVS is sensitive to unique foods and so you can not define any certain foods which trigger CVS in general.

- **Psychological stress.** Psychological stress can also trigger a CVS episode. If you suffer from mental stress or something keeps worrying you, there is a high chance that you are suffering from psychological stress. You should try to get psychological stress-management counseling which will help you control the level of stress and not get anxious. Once you are in control of it, you can avoid the triggering of CVS episodes.

- **Motion sickness.** In some people, motion sickness is induced by something as simple as traveling for a few miles in a car. This can cause nausea and vomiting and can lead to a CVS attack. There is also the possibility that you are not always motion-sick and it's only sometimes that traveling makes you feel nauseated. If that is the case, you should avoid traveling at times when you feel motion-sick. This will help you avoid CVS episodes.

- **Wrong dietary habits.** These include eating too much or eating just before you go to bed. If you have CVS and you don't take care of your dietary habits, you may end up getting CVS attacks quite frequently. So it's really important that you regulate your diet, take it on proper time and do not overdo it.

Three: Common symptoms and signs of CVS

If you are suffering from CVS, the most common symptom that you will face is nausea. You will feel very nauseated and this can lead to episodes of vomiting. Sometimes, the episodes may last for 24 hours. Typically, an episode starts early in the morning or when you wake up. The first hour is the hardest because you experience excessive vomiting. You may experience vomiting five to six times during the first hour. After the first hour, the frequency of vomiting may begin to decline. After 24 hours, the feeling of nausea may go away and vomiting stops. Sometimes the episode may be longer than 1 day. It may last up to four days and in some cases, up to ten days. Once the episode ends, it may take you a few hours to get back to normal and be able to eat and drink. The condition may return after a few days or weeks without any warning.

According to most patients, nausea is also the most distressing symptom of CVS. When it lasts for hours, it can be extremely annoying. You may find yourself unable to do anything. The symptom ends only when the episode of vomiting ends, which is usually after a total of 24 hours.

- Abdominal pain. About 80% of CVS patients suffer from abdominal pain. In some cases, you may start experiencing abdominal pain just before an episode starts. So this pain can be a signal of a CVS attack about to happen and if you immediately take some medicine to treat the abdominal pain, you may be able to stop the CVS attack.

- The feelings of nausea and the vomiting that this nausea causes may severely affect your social life. At some random days, without any warning, when the episode starts, you may have to take an absent from work and stay at home. You may miss a birthday or a party because of the symptoms. Such things can adversely affect your social life if you don't tackle it correctly. For example, if your friends and colleagues at work are aware of this condition and they know that you may have to be absent any time without any forewarning, they will understand when your CVS episodes start.

- One-third of CVS patients suffer from symptoms such as headache, fever and diarrhea. If you suffer from diarrhea together with CVS, this can be quite dangerous because you run a high risk of dehydration.

- Lethargy. You may feel lazy and lethargic when an episode of CVS starts. You may also feel weak due to excessive vomiting which can make your body deficient of water and nutrients. In some cases the lethargy may be so thorough that a person may seem to be in a coma and may be unable to walk or talk normally.

- Salivation. You may suffer from excessive salivation. This, added to the feeling of nausea, can make you feel very irritated and annoyed.

- Photophobia. You may want to turn off all the lights and the TV when the CVS episodes start. A patient who suffers from migraine also experiences photophobia. Because of this, doctors believe that there is a link between migraine and CVS.

- Phonophobia. Phonophobia is a fear for loud voices. When you suffer from CVS, you may want everyone to be silent. Even the slight sounds, such as the sound of the revolving of a fan, may make you feel very irritated.

- Vertigo. This is a condition in which you may feel that you are moving even when you are stationary. The vestibular system in the ear helps you balance yourself and walk steadily. But this system may malfunction during CVS and you may feel a loss of balance when walking.

- Episodes of vomiting. If these episodes are triggered by some sort of excitement or due to a special diet, such as a high-protein meal, there is a very high chance that you are suffering from CVS. They may be triggered by both happy and worrisome excitements. For example, if you are excited about something because it makes you nervous, it can lead to a CVS attack. At the same time, if you are very happy and excited about something, for instance a promotion, even that can cause a CVS attack. Such triggers are clear symptoms that you have CVS.

- Abnormal neurologic symptoms. These include sudden mood swings and changes in mental health, abnormal movements of the eye-ball and talking or walking awkwardly at times.

- A worsening of vomiting episodes. In many cases, CVS no longer is cyclic. It can take up a pattern where you continuously can suffer from this condition any time.

- Ataxia. Ataxia results in an abnormal coordination of the muscles so that if you suffer from it, you may make clumsy movements without realizing it.

- Dystonia. This causes the twisting of the muscles and abnormal postures.

- Confusion. This is a result of rapidly changing mental status you may experience during CVS episodes.

- Drooling. You may experience excessive saliva production which may cause drooling.

There are a number of things that may make your symptoms worse. 68% of the families of CVS patients say that certain things or events make the CVS symptoms grow severe. In about 41% of the patients, infections make the CVS symptoms worse – for example, an infection of the air-passage near the nose called sinusitis is a common trigger for CVS attacks. In a large number of patients, psychological stress also triggers the symptoms. For this reason, if you are suffering from CVS, you should try to keep a cool head and not get stressed or anxious over something. You should try not to worry too much about anything or it can trigger an episode of CVS. If you continue to have psychological stress which triggers CVS episodes, you should seek psychological counseling for stress management.

You should know that not only negative but also positive kind of excitement can trigger an episode of CVS. For example, if you are at a birthday or a party or if you are very happy over something, there is a high chance that this may trigger CVS symptoms. According to research, a positive form of excitement more often triggers the symptoms than the negative form of excitement.

A number of food products such as chocolate and cheese can also worsen the symptoms of CVS. This may be different for different people. For example, some person's CVS may be triggered when he eats cheese while your CVS may be triggered by some other food. You'll learn what kind of foods trigger the attack when you experience a CVS episode after eating it.

Other factors that may trigger CVS symptoms include insomnia (lack of sleep), motion sickness and vomiting due to some other reasons. These may include over-eating and being careless about your dietary habits which can result in vomiting. This can then trigger a CVS attack which may results in more vomiting.

Four: Diagnosis

The symptoms of CVS are similar to the symptoms of a number of other diseases. So you have to be careful in having it diagnosed correctly. Your doctor will first diagnose you for a number of other conditions, related to diseases of stomach and intestine, with similar symptoms. Once he is sure that you are not suffering from any of them, he will treat you for CVS.

You should also tell your doctor about medical history in detail. This will help him decide if your symptoms are a result of some other condition or if they really are a result of CVS. In some cases, the doctor will ask you to go back and come again if a CVS episode occurs. This is usually done to confirm that there is a cyclic nature to your condition as happens in CVS. Normally, four to five episodes confirm that a patient is suffering from cyclic vomiting syndrome.

The other conditions which have similar symptoms as CVS are:

- Gastrointestinal disorder which means any disorder of the esophagus, stomach or the intestines. Such disorders can induce nausea and cause vomiting.

- Gastroesophageal reflux disease (GERD). In this condition, the acid produced by the stomach rises up through the esophagus. This can cause a feeling of burning in the chest and you may experience acidic vomits.

- Peptic ulcers. In such disorders, the stomach malfunctions and the acids produced by the stomach can harm the lining of the stomach and the duodenum. Peptic ulcers may also be a result of a bacterial infection of the stomach or the intestines, such as helicobacter pylori. They can cause vomiting, with the vomits containing stomach acids. This is exactly the case in CVS vomits too and so, both conditions have a lot of common symptoms.

- Inflammatory bowel diseases. Inflammatory bowel diseases usually affect the small intestine. A common known inflammatory bowel disease is Crohn's disease. In this condition, any part of the passage of the food, from your mouth to the end of large intestine, may get affected. The symptoms may be abdominal pain, diarrhea, loss of weight and vomiting.

- Intestinal obstruction. It can be caused by tumors in your intestine. The intestine gets blocked due to it.

- Hirschsprung's disease. In this condition, you may suffer from constipation, vomiting and abdominal pain and it is more common in children than adults.

- Migraine. It can be pain in the head, causing severe headache. Or an abdominal migraine, causing severe pain in the stomach. Like CVS, these two types of migraine have symptoms which start very suddenly and end abruptly and after they end, the patient feels perfectly normal until the next cycle of symptoms begins. Migraine and CVS are also linked because children who have migraine in their family often suffer from CVS. So it is important for the doctor to make sure that he diagnosed correctly whether you are suffering from CVS or migraine. This takes time and will need extensive diagnosis and a number of tests which are listed below.

Tests for CVS:

To diagnose CVS correctly and to rule out the possibilities of other diseases with similar symptoms, you may have to go through the following tests:

- A small-bowel follow-through (SMFT) radiography. This is a radiologic scan of the small intestine. This is done to check whether or not you are suffering from an intestinal disease.

Small bowel follow-through

Diagnostics

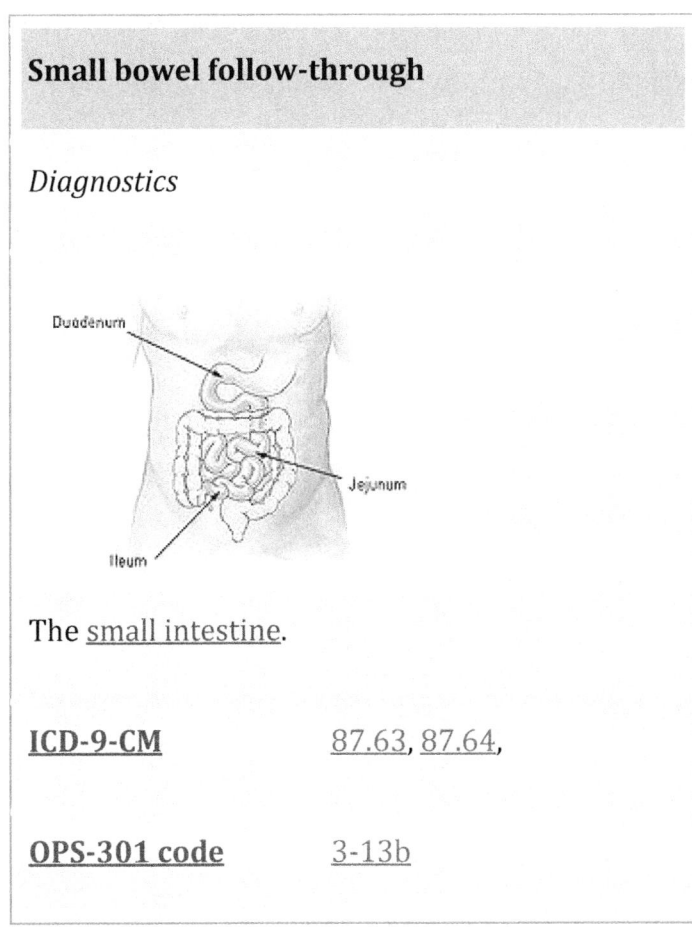

The small intestine.

ICD-9-CM   87.63, 87.64,

OPS-301 code   3-13b

Diagnostics

3-13b The small intestine.

A small bowel follow-through, also called small bowel series, is a radiologic examination of the small intestine from the distal duodenum/duodenojejunal junction to the ileocecal valve.

An X-ray examination of the most proximal small bowel (duodenum) is typically done together with an examination of the esophagus and stomach and is called an upper GI series.

Procedure

Person drinks radio-opaque contrast.
X-ray images of abdomen are made at timed intervals.

Indications

Pathology of the small bowel is uncommon. Therefore, upper GI and lower GI endoscopy is often done prior to small bowel follow-through.

Categorically, the indications are:
Negative upper endoscopy and negative lower endoscopy
Investigation of a small bowel abnormality found on other medical imaging

Specific indications

Suspected small bowel neoplasm, e.g. small bowel cancer

Hematochezia

Positive fecal occult blood test

Suspected small bowel obstruction that has been managed conservatively

Inflammatory bowel disease (Crohn's disease

Upper GI series, also upper gastrointestinal (GI) tract radiography, is a radiologic examination of the upper gastrointestinal tract. It consists of a series of X-ray images of the esophagus, stomach and duodenum. The most common use for this medical testing is to look for signs of ulcers, acid reflux disease, uncontrollable vomiting, or unexplained blood in the stools (hematochezia or positive fecal occult blood).

Application / Preparation

When the patient needs to undertake an upper GI, he or she is asked to take a fast on the previous day, depending on what the doctor wishes the patient to take or what might be the needed for this testing. Normally, the patient must avoid solid food for up to eight hours prior to the appointment and avoid any type of consumable, including water, three hours prior to the testing.

Process

This is a non-invasive test, consisting of an X-ray. In the X-ray room, the patient is given two medications to drink that help improve the quality of the resulting X-rays. The patient may also be administered glucagon, a pancreatic hormone that is injected intravenously. The first drink is very carbonated, made from baking-soda crystals which expands the stomach by causing gas to build in the stomach. The second drink is a contrast agent, typically a thick, chalky liquid containing a barium salt. (This test is sometimes called a barium swallow.) The barium outlines the stomach on the X-rays, helping the doctor find tumors or other abnormal areas.

The patient then has X-rays taken. The doctors usually take a series of pictures with the patient in a number of different positions to capture different poses and views of the digestive system. Normally the patient needs to hold their breath to avoid the pictures from blurring and causing unneeded challenges in diagnosing the illness.

During the test, the doctor may pump air into the stomach to make features such as small tumors easier to see.

After the test

Patients may feel nauseated immediately after drinking the barium. This is common and may last up to 72 hours following the test. Patients may eat as normal after the procedure but it is important to drink a lot of water to allow the barium to pass through the body more easily. Constipation is common but diarrhea will affect some patients. Another common side effect is the bleaching of solid waste matter; this may last up to 48 hours.

Ephagogastroduodenoscopy. It is the examination of the stomach and the starting part of the small intestine (duodenum) with the help of the endoscope, a medical instrument. Stomach and intestinal diseases are collectively called gastrointestinal diseases or GI diseases. This examination is does to confirm you are not suffering from any GI problems.

Esophagogastroduodenoscopy

Intervention

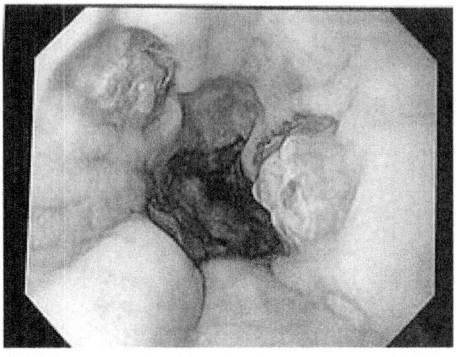

Endoscopic still of esophageal ulcers seen after banding of esophageal varices, at time of esophagogastroduodenosocopy

ICD-9-CM	45.13
MeSH	D016145
OPS-301 code:	1-631, 1-632

In medicine (gastroenterology), **esophagogastroduodenoscopy** is a diagnostic endoscopic procedure that visualizes the upper part of the gastrointestinal tract up to the duodenum. It is considered a minimally invasive procedure since it does not require an incision into one of the major body cavities and does not require any significant recovery after the procedure (unless sedation or anesthesia has been used). A sore throat is also common.[1][2][3]

Alternative names

Esophagogastroduodenoscopy may be abbreviated **EGD**, or **OGD** if one uses the British spelling **oesophagogastroduodenoscopy**. It is also called **upper GI endoscopy** (UGIE), **gastroscopy** or simply endoscopy (since it is the most commonly performed type of endoscopy, the ambiguous term 'endoscopy' refers to EGD by default).

Indications

Diagnostic

- Unexplained anemia (usually along with a colonoscopy)
- Upper gastrointestinal bleeding as evidenced by hematemesis or melena
- Persistent dyspepsia in patients over the age of 45 years

- Heartburn and chronic acid reflux - this can lead to a precancerous lesion called Barrett's esophagus
- Persistent vomiting
- Dysphagia - difficulty in swallowing
- Odynophagia - painful swallowing
- **Surveillance**

- Surveillance of Barrett's esophagus
- Surveillance of gastric ulcer or duodenal ulcer
- Occasionally after gastric surgery
- **Confirmation of diagnosis/biopsy**

- Abnormal barium swallow or barium meal
- Confirmation of celiac disease (via biopsy)
- **Therapeutic**

- Treatment (banding/sclerotherapy) of esophageal varices
- Injection therapy (e.g. epinephrine in bleeding lesions)
- Cutting off of larger pieces of tissue with a snare device (e.g. polyps, endoscopic mucosal resection)
- Application of cautery to tissues

- Removal of foreign bodies (e.g. food) that have been ingested
- Tamponade of bleeding esophageal varices with a balloon
- Application of photodynamic therapy for treatment of esophageal malignancies
- Endoscopic drainage of pancreatic pseudocyst
- Tightening the lower esophageal sphincter
- Dilating or stenting of stenosis or achalasia
- Percutaneous endoscopic gastrostomy (feeding tube placement)
- Endoscopic retrograde cholangiopancreatography (ERCP) combines EGD with fluoroscopy
- Endoscopic ultrasound (EUS) combines EGD with 5–12 MHz ultrasound imaging
- **Newer interventions**
- Endoscopic trans-gastric laparoscopy
- Placement of gastric balloons in bariatric surgery

Equipment

- Endoscope

- Non-coaxial optic fiber system to carry light to the tip of the endoscope
- A chip camera at the tip of the endoscope - this has now replaced the coaxial optic fibers of older scopes that were prone to damage and consequent loss of picture quality
- Irrigation channel to clean the lens
- Suction/Insufflation/Working channels - these may be in the form of one or more channels
- Control handle - this houses the controls
- Stack
  - Light source
  - Insufflator
  - Suction
  - Electrosurgical unit
  - Video recorder/photo printer
- Instruments
  - Biopsy forceps
  - Snares
  - Injecting needles

Procedure

The patient is kept NPO (Nil per os) or NBM (Nothing By Mouth) that is, told not to eat, for at least 4–6 hours before the procedure. Most patients tolerate the procedure with only topical anesthesia of the oropharynx using lidocaine spray. However, some patients may need sedation and the very anxious/agitated patient may even need a general anesthetic. Informed consent is obtained before the procedure. The main risks are bleeding and perforation. The risk is increased when a biopsy or other intervention is performed.

The patient lies on his/her left side with the head resting comfortably on a pillow. A mouth-guard is placed between the teeth to prevent the patient from biting on the endoscope. The endoscope is then passed over the tongue and into the oropharynx. This is the most uncomfortable stage for the patient. Quick and gentle manipulation under vision guides the endoscope into the esophagus. The endoscope is gradually advanced down the esophagus making note of any pathology. Excessive insufflation of the stomach is avoided at this stage. The endoscope is quickly passed through the stomach and through the pylorus to examine the first and second parts of the duodenum. Once this has been completed, the endoscope is withdrawn into the stomach and a more thorough examination is performed including a J-maneuver. This involves retroflexing the tip of the scope so it resembles a 'J' shape in order to examine the fundus and gastroesophageal junction. Any additional procedures are performed at this stage. The air in the stomach is aspirated before removing the endoscope.

Still photographs can be made during the procedure and later shown to the patient to help explain any findings.

In its most basic use, the endoscope is used to *inspect* the internal anatomy of the digestive tract. Often inspection alone is sufficient, but biopsy is a very valuable adjunct to endoscopy. Small biopsies can be made with a pincer (biopsy forceps) which is passed through the scope and allows sampling of 1 to 3 mm pieces of tissue under direct vision. The intestinal mucosa heals quickly from such biopsies.

Biopsy allows the pathologist to render an opinion on later histologic examination of the biopsy tissue with light microscopy and/or immunohistochemistry.

Biopsied material can also be tested on urease to identify *Helicobacter pylori*.

Complications

The complication rate is about 1 in 1000. They include:

- aspiration, causing aspiration pneumonia
- bleeding
- perforation
- cardiopulmonary problems

Limitations

Problems of gastrointestinal *function* are usually not well diagnosed by endoscopy since *motion* or *secretion* of the gastrointestinal tract are not easily inspected by EGD. Nonetheless, findings such as excess fluid or poor motion of gut during endoscopy can be suggestive of disorders of function. Irritable bowel syndrome and functional dyspepsia is not diagnosed with EGD, but EGD may be helpful in excluding other diseases that mimic these common disorders.

Additional images

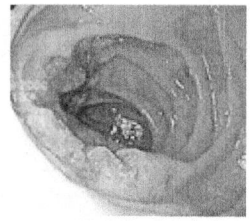

- Endoscopic image of adenocarcinoma of duodenumseen in the post-bulbar duodenum.

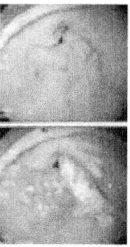

- Endoscopic image of gastric antral vascular ectasia seen as a radial pattern around thepylorus before (top) and after (bottom) treatment with argon plasma coagulation

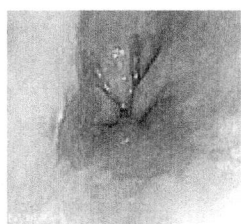

Endoscopic image of Barrett's esophagus, which is the area of red mucosa projecting like a tongue.

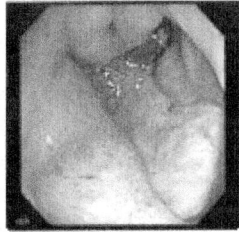

Deep gastric ulcer

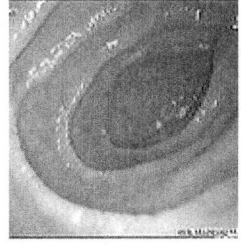

Endoscopic still of duodenum of patient with celiac disease showing scalloping of folds.

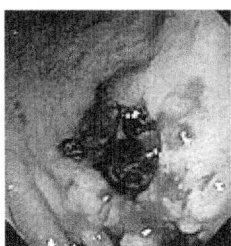

Gastric ulcer in antrum of stomach with overlying clot due to gastric lymphoma.

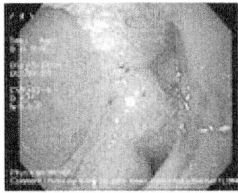

Endoscopic image of a posterior wall duodenal ulcer with a clean base, which is a common cause of upper GI hemorrhage.

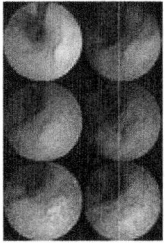

Endoscopic images of an early stage stomach cancer. 0-IIa, tub1. Left column: Normal light. Right column: computed image enhanced(FICE). First row: Normal. Second row:Acetate stained. Third row: Acetate-indigocarmine mixture(AIM) stained.

Abdominal ultrasonography. Ultrasound waves from a machine are used to visualize the inner structure of your abdomen. This test is used to diagnose any abnormalities that may occur in your internal organs or the abdominal region.

Abdominal ultrasonography

Intervention

ICD-9-CM	88.76
OPS-301 code:	3-059

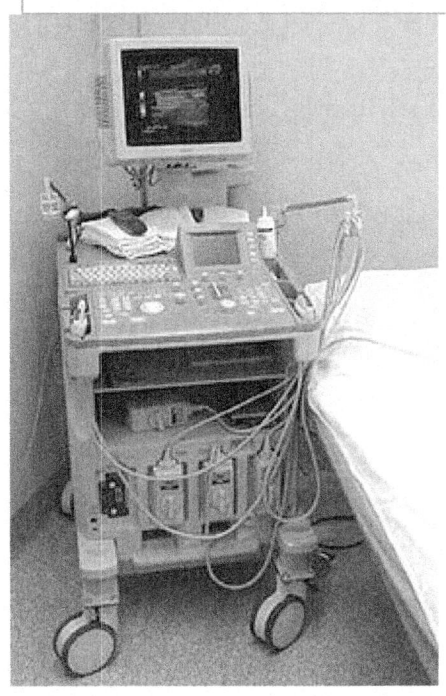

Medical ultrasound equipment which can be used for abdominal ultrasonography.

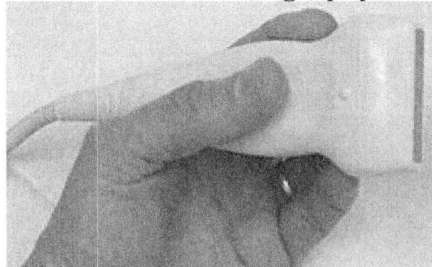

Ultrasound probe placed on the abdominal wall.

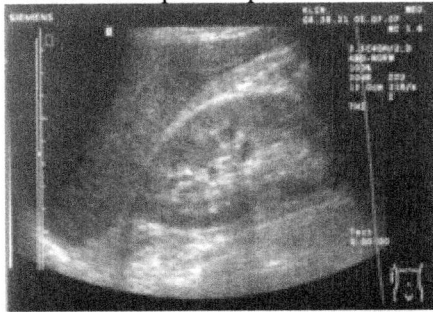

Ultrasound scan of a kidney (right side).

Abdominal ultrasonography (also called **abdominal ultrasound imaging** or **abdominal sonography**) is a form of medical ultrasonography (medical application of ultrasound technology) to visualise abdominal anatomical structures. It uses transmission and reflection of ultrasound waves to visualise internal organs through the abdominal wall (with the help of gel which helps transmission of the sound waves). For this reason, the procedure is also called a **transabdominal ultrasound**, in contrast with endoscopic ultrasound, the latter combining ultrasound with endoscopy through visualize internal structures from within hollow organs.

Abdominal ultrasound examinations are performed by gastroenterologists or certain other specialists in internal medicine, radiologists or sonographers trained for this procedure.

Usage

Abdominal ultrasound can be used to diagnose abnormalities in various internal organs, such as the kidneys,[1] liver, gallbladder, pancreas, spleen and a bdominal aorta. If Doppler imaging is added, the blood flow inside blood vessels can be evaluated as well (for example, to look for renal artery stenosis).

Through the abdominal wall, organs inside the pelvis can be seen, such as the as urinary bladder or the ovaries and uterus in women. Because water is an excellent conductor for ultrasound waves, visualizing these structures often requires a well-filled urinary bladder (this means the patients has to drink plenty of water before the examination).

Abdominal ultrasound is commonly used in the setting of abdominal pain or an acute abdomen (sudden and/or severe abdominal pain syndrome in which surgical intervention might be necessary), in which it can diagnose appendicitis orcholecystitis.

In patients with deranged liver function tests, ultrasound may show increased liver size (hepatomegaly), increased reflectiveness (which might, for example, indicate cholestasis), gallbladder or bile duct diseases, or a tumor in the liver. The same is true for patients with an abnormal kidney function or pancreatic enzymes(pancreatic amylase and pancreatic lipase), in which ultrasound can be used for additional anatomical information.

Ultrasound can also be used if there is suspicion of enlargement of one or more organs, such as used in screening for abdominal aortic aneurysm, investigation for splenomegaly or urinary retention.

Ultrasound imaging is useful for detecting stones, for example kidney stones or gallstones, because they create a clearly visible ultrasound shadow behind the stone.

Ultrasonography can be used to guide procedures such as treatment for kidney stones with Extracorporeal shock wave lithotripsy,
needle biopsies or paracentesis (needle drainage of free fluid inside the abdominal cavity).

Advantages and disadvantages

Advantages of ultrasound imaging of abdominal structures are that the procedure can be performed quickly, bed-side, involves no exposure to X-rays (which makes it useful in pregnant patients, for example) and is inexpensive compared to other often-used techniques such as computed tomography (CT scan) of the abdomen. Disadvantages are troublesome imaging if a lot of gas is present inside the bowels, if there is a lot of abdominal fat, and that the quality of the imaging depends on the experience of the person performing it.

The imaging occurs real-time and without sedation, so that the influence of movements can be assessed quickly. For example, by pressing the ultrasound probe against the gallbladder, a radiological Murphy's sign can be elicited.

Other possible tests:

- **Gastric emptying scan (GES).** This is a test that lasts from 90 minutes to up to six hours. You will be given specific foods to eat after which the test will be done. The test is aimed at checking whether or not the food passes normally through the food passage of the body, including the stomach and the intestines. The test tells whether or not there are any intestinal blockages.
- **Sinus CT scan.** Sinuses are pockets of air in your head. These may fill up with mucus and cause an infection. A CT scan is a computerized topography scan which creates a three-dimensional image of an object. A CT scan on the sinus is used to

detect whether or not you are suffering from a sinusitis (sinus infection).

- **A brain MRI** (magnetic resonance imaging). This test is used to produce detailed images of the brain. The test is done so as to ensure that you don't have any brain-related problems or any malfunctioning of the nervous system.

- **Renal ultrasonography.** This is an ultrasound imaging of the kidneys. This test is done to check if your kidneys malfunction and if, as a result, the urine produced by your body is not normally excreted.

- **Psychological evaluation tests.** These are done to check your mental health and to see if you are suffering from a case of anxiety or stress. At times, psychological problems can lead to eating disorders which can cause abnormal functioning of the stomach. So a psychological evaluation is very important so as to ensure that your CVS is not actually a stomach-problem with similar symptoms.

There are a lot of diseases which have similar symptoms as GVS. It can be quite difficult for the doctor to diagnose CVS correctly. You will have to undergo a number of tests to make sure that you don't have any other gastrointestinal diseases. This may take some time and can prove to be somewhat expensive. The doctor may also ask you to come back again in a few days after taking these tests. This is usually done to ensure that there is a cyclic nature to your vomiting episodes and that they appear again and again. If the vomiting episode occurred only once, the doctor will know that it isn't CVS. But if it happened more than once, you and your doctor will know that it's cyclic, which is a clear symptom of CVS.

Five: Treatment

Since no definite cause for CVS is known, there is no definite treatment known for the condition. So the doctors try to take a general approach which is aimed at avoiding the symptoms. The following five strategies are most commonly used:

- Trying to avoid the CVS episodes as much as possible. This can be done by first determining what triggers your CVS episodes. It can be a certain food, motion sickness, excitement, psychological stress or any other factor. You should identify that factor and then try to avoid it as much as possible.

- Prophylactic pharmacotherapy. This is used to treat migraine headaches. The main medications used in this therapy are erythromycin, propranolol, cyproheptadine and amitriptyline.

- Abortive therapy. This therapy is used to stop CVS symptoms from growing worse. In such cases where abortive therapy doesn't improve the condition, medications such as a combination of chlorpromazine and diphenhydramine or lorazepam and ondansetron may be helpful in reducing the intensity of a vomiting episode.

- Supportive care when an episode occurs. This includes being ready to treat the main symptoms of the episode such as nausea, vomiting etc.

- Family support. If you are suffering from CVS, your social life is greatly affected and you may find yourself unable to go to work on days when the CVS episodes occur. Also, you may feel very irritated and annoyed due to the feeling of nausea that accompanies CVS episodes. During all this, you will need family support to help you with this condition and support you while it lasts. Family support is very important because it helps you stabilize your social life despite CVS.

Pharmacologic therapy is also used sometimes to reduce the frequency of vomiting or to you help you control the episodes of vomiting and avoid them. You may drink water to dilute the acid present in the vomit. This will make vomiting less bitter. But drinking water can lead to more vomiting and an increased feeling of nausea. If the episode lasts longer, you body may run the risk of dehydration because you lose a lot of water through vomiting. At such a time, you may need IV fluids to be supplied to your body or your body will grow very weak.

In some patients, CVS episodes occur when they take certain diets. For example, you may trigger a CVS episode if you take chocolate or cheese or certain foods specific to you. In that case, you should try to avoid such foods. By just avoiding eating such foods, you may be successful in preventing any CVS attacks.

In some cases, the main cause that leads to CVS episodes is psychological. If you are facing psychological stress, that may lead to a CVS episode. In such a case, you should consult a psychiatrist who will help you learn techniques through which you will be able to tackle mental stress and avoid the CVS attack. Medications usually suggested for CVS episodes which are a result of psychological stress are lorazepam or diazepam.

Some CVS triggers are common daily-life happenings and simply can't be avoided. For example, if your CVS episode is triggered by a ride in a car which results in nausea and leads to vomiting, it can be very hard for you to avoid it. Similarly, common bacterial infections can also trigger CVS symptoms. The good news for you is that a majority of CVS patients, about 70%, are able to decrease the intensity and frequency of CVS episodes with a change in their lifestyles. For instance, if your CVS is triggered by certain foods, you can rule them out of your diet. If they are a result of psychological stress, you can regularly see a psychiatrist and take lessons at stress management. Consultation has also proved to be really helpful in getting rid of CVS symptoms.

If your CVS results in severe symptoms and disables you physically in some way, for example leaving you unable to walk or talk, you should take some medications on regular basis to treat these symptoms. These include antimigraine drugs if your symptoms are caused by migraine; anticonvulsants and neuroleptics. If someone in your family suffers from migraine, or if you suffer from migraine, there is a very high chance that you may be able to control the CVS episodes with the help of antimigraine drugs.

In children younger than 5 years, cyproheptadine is recommended as a medication that reduces the frequency and severity of the episodes. But a side-effect of cyproheptadine is that it increases the appetite of the user and can result in an increase in the weight of the child. Other episodes which are used for the same purpose in older patients are amitriptyline, cyproheptadine and propranolol. Phenobarbital, another medication, is also used for the treatment of CVS episodes with a success rate of 79%. Erythromycin has a success rate of 75%.

Alternative Therapies

Alternative therapies that may alleviate CVS symptoms include meditation and yoga. You may be surprised to learn that many yoga studios offer yoga to children. There's one in my hometown that even caters to toddlers.

Meditation

Meditation is known to be a very powerful tool to counter pain with. At first, it certainly will seem very hard but with practice, if can become a powerful tool to combat pain. Meditation is a mind-body practice in complementary and alternative medicine (CAM). There are many types of meditation, most of which originated in ancient religious and spiritual traditions. Generally, a person who is meditating uses certain techniques, such as a specific posture, focused attention, and an open attitude toward distractions. Meditation may be practiced for many reasons, such as to increase calmness and physical relaxation, to improve psychological balance, to cope with illness, or to enhance overall health and well-being. This Backgrounder provides a general introduction to meditation and suggests some resources for more information.

People practice meditation for a number of health-related purposes.

It is not fully known what changes occur in the body during meditation; whether they influence health; and, if so, how. Research is under way to find out more about meditation's effects, how it works, and diseases and conditions for which it may be most helpful.

Tell your health care providers about any complementary and alternative practices you use. Give them a full picture of what you do to manage your health. This will help ensure coordinated and safe care.

The term meditation refers to a group of techniques, such as mantra meditation, relaxation response, mindfulness meditation, and Zen Buddhist meditation. Most meditative techniques started in Eastern religious or spiritual traditions. These techniques have been used by many different cultures throughout the world for thousands of years. Today, many people use meditation outside of its traditional religious or cultural settings, for health and well-being.

In meditation, a person learns to focus attention. Some forms of meditation instruct the practitioner to become mindful of thoughts, feelings, and sensations and to observe them in a nonjudgmental way. This practice is believed to result in a state of greater calmness and physical relaxation, and psychological balance. Practicing meditation can change how a person relates to the flow of emotions and thoughts.

Most types of meditation have four elements in common:

A quiet location. Meditation is usually practiced in a quiet place with as few distractions as possible. This can be particularly helpful for beginners.

A specific, comfortable posture. Depending on the type being practiced, meditation can be done while sitting, lying down, standing, walking, or in other positions.

A focus of attention. Focusing one's attention is usually a part of meditation. For example, the meditator may focus on a mantra (a specially chosen word or set of words), an object, or the sensations of the breath. Some forms of meditation involve paying attention to whatever is the dominant content of consciousness.

An open attitude. Having an open attitude during meditation means letting distractions come and go naturally without judging them. When the attention goes to distracting or wandering thoughts, they are not suppressed; instead, the meditator gently brings attention back to the focus. In some types of meditation, the meditator learns to "observe" thoughts and emotions while meditating.

Meditation used as CAM is a type of mind-body medicine. Generally, mind-body medicine focuses on:

The interactions among the brain/mind, the rest of the body, and behavior.

The ways in which emotional, mental, social, spiritual, and behavioral factors can directly affect health.

Uses of Meditation for Health in the United States

A 2007 national Government survey that asked about CAM use in a sample of 23,393 U.S. adults found that 9.4 percent of respondents (representing more than 20 million people) had used meditation in the past 12 months—compared with 7.6 percent of respondents (representing more than 15 million people) in a similar survey conducted in 2002. The 2007 survey also asked about CAM use in a sample of 9,417 children; 1 percent (representing 725,000 children) had used meditation in the past 12 months.

People use meditation for various health problems, such as:

Anxiety

Pain

Depression

Stress

Insomnia

Physical or emotional symptoms that may be associated with chronic illnesses (such as heart disease, HIV/AIDS, and cancer) and their treatment.

Meditation is also used for overall wellness.

Examples of Meditation Practices

Mindfulness meditation and Transcendental Meditation (also known as TM) are two common forms of meditation. NCCAM-sponsored research projects are studying both types of meditation.

Mindfulness meditation is an essential component of Buddhism. In one common form of mindfulness meditation, the meditator is taught to bring attention to the sensation of the flow of the breath in and out of the body. The meditator learns to focus attention on what is being experienced, without reacting to or judging it. This is seen as helping the meditator learn to experience thoughts and emotions in normal daily life with greater balance and acceptance.

The TM technique is derived from Hindu traditions. It uses a mantra (a word, sound, or phrase repeated silently) to prevent distracting thoughts from entering the mind. The goal of TM is to achieve a state of relaxed awareness.

How Meditation Might Work

Practicing meditation has been shown to induce some changes in the body. By learning more about what goes on in the body during meditation, researchers hope to be able to identify diseases or conditions for which meditation might be useful.

Some types of meditation might work by affecting the autonomic (involuntary) nervous system. This system regulates many organs and muscles, controlling functions such as heartbeat, sweating, breathing, and digestion. It has two major parts:

The sympathetic nervous system helps mobilize the body for action. When a person is under stress, it produces the "fight-or-flight response": the heart rate and breathing rate go up and blood vessels narrow (restricting the flow of blood).

The parasympathetic nervous system causes the heart rate and breathing rate to slow down, the blood vessels to dilate (improving blood flow), and the flow of digestive juices increases.

It is thought that some types of meditation might work by reducing activity in the sympathetic nervous system and increasing activity in the parasympathetic nervous system.

In one area of research, scientists are using sophisticated tools to determine whether meditation is associated with significant changes in brain function. A number of researchers believe that these changes account for many of meditation's effects.

It is also possible that practicing meditation may work by improving the mind's ability to pay attention. Since attention is involved in performing everyday tasks and regulating mood, meditation might lead to other benefits.

A 2007 NCCAM-funded review of the scientific literature found some evidence suggesting that meditation is associated with potentially beneficial health effects. However, the overall evidence was inconclusive. The reviewers concluded that future research needs to be more rigorous before firm conclusions can be drawn.

Side Effects and Risks

Meditation is considered to be safe for healthy people. There have been rare reports that meditation could cause or worsen symptoms in people who have certain psychiatric problems, but this question has not been fully researched. People with physical limitations may not be able to participate in certain meditative practices involving physical movement. Individuals with existing mental or physical health conditions should speak with their health care providers prior to starting a meditative practice and make their meditation instructor aware of their condition.

If You Are Thinking About Using Meditation Practices

Do not use meditation as a replacement for conventional care or as a reason to postpone seeing a doctor about a medical problem.

Ask about the training and experience of the meditation instructor you are considering.

Look for published research studies on meditation for the health condition in which you are interested.

Tell all your health care providers about any complementary and alternative practices you use. Give them a full picture of what you do to manage your health. This will help ensure coordinated and safe care. For tips about talking with your health care providers about CAM, see NCCAM's Time to Talk campaign at http://nccam.nih.gov/timetotalk/.

NCCAM-Supported Research

Some recent NCCAM-supported studies have been investigating meditation for:

Relieving stress in caregivers for elderly patients with dementia

Reducing the frequency and intensity of hot flashes in menopausal women

Relieving symptoms of chronic back pain

Yoga

Yoga is a mind-body practice in complementary and alternative medicine (CAM) with origins in ancient Indian philosophy. The various styles of yoga that people use for health purposes typically combine physical postures, breathing techniques, and meditation or relaxation. There are numerous schools of yoga. Hatha yoga, the most commonly practiced in the United States and Europe, emphasizes postures (asanas) and breathing exercises (pranayama). Some of the major styles of hatha yoga include Iyengar, Ashtanga, Vini, Kundalini, and Bikram yoga. People use yoga for a variety of conditions and to achieve fitness and relaxation.

The 2007 National Health Interview Survey found that yoga is one of the top 10 CAM modalities used among U.S. adults. An estimated 6 percent of adults used yoga for health purposes in the previous 12 months.

People use yoga for a variety of health conditions and to achieve fitness and relaxation.

It is not fully known what changes occur in the body during yoga; whether they influence health; and if so, how. There is, however, growing evidence to suggest that yoga works to enhance stress-coping mechanisms and mind-body awareness. Research is under way to find out more about yoga's effects, and the diseases and conditions for which it may be most helpful.

Tell your health care providers about any complementary and alternative practices you use. Give them a full picture of what you do to manage your health. This will help ensure coordinated and safe care.

Overview

Yoga in its full form combines physical postures, breathing exercises, meditation, and a distinct philosophy. Yoga is intended to increase relaxation and balance the mind, body, and the spirit.

Early written descriptions of yoga are in Sanskrit, the classical language of India. The word "yoga" comes from the Sanskrit word yuj, which means "yoke or union." It is believed that this describes the union between the mind and the body. The first known text, The Yoga Sutras, was written more than 2,000 years ago, although yoga may have been practiced as early as 5,000 years ago. Yoga was originally developed as a method of discipline and attitudes to help people reach spiritual enlightenment. The Sutras outline eight limbs or foundations of yoga practice that serve as spiritual guidelines:

> yama (moral behavior)
>
> niyama (healthy habits)
>
> asana (physical postures)
>
> pranayama (breathing exercises)
>
> pratyahara (sense withdrawal)
>
> dharana (concentration)
>
> dhyana (contemplation)
>
> samadhi (higher consciousness)

The numerous schools of yoga incorporate these eight limbs in varying proportions. Hatha yoga, the most commonly practiced in the United States and Europe, emphasizes two of the eight limbs: postures (asanas) and breathing exercises (pranayama). Some of the major styles of hatha yoga include Ananda, Anusara, Ashtanga, Bikram, Iyengar, Kripalu, Kundalini, and Viniyoga.

Use of Yoga for Health in the United States

According to the 2007 National Health Interview Survey (NHIS), which included a comprehensive survey of

CAM use by Americans, yoga is one of the top 10 CAM modalities used. More than 13 million adults had used yoga in the previous year, and between the 2002 and 2007 NHIS, use of yoga among adults increased by 1 percent (or approximately 3 million people). The 2007 survey also found that more than 1.5 million children used yoga in the previous year.

People use yoga for a variety of health conditions including anxiety disorders or stress, asthma, high blood pressure, and depression. People also use yoga as part of a general health regimen—to achieve physical fitness and to relax.

The Status of Yoga Research

Research suggests that yoga might:

Improve mood and sense of well-being

Counteract stress

Reduce heart rate and blood pressure

Increase lung capacity

Improve muscle relaxation and body composition

Help with conditions such as anxiety, depression, and insomnia

Improve overall physical fitness, strength, and flexibility

Positively affect levels of certain brain or blood chemicals.

More well-designed studies are needed before definitive conclusions can be drawn about yoga's use for specific health conditions.

Side Effects and Risks

Yoga is generally considered to be safe in healthy people when practiced appropriately. Studies have found it to be well tolerated, with few side effects.

People with certain medical conditions should not use some yoga practices. For example, people with disc disease of the spine, extremely high or low blood pressure, glaucoma, retinal detachment, fragile or atherosclerotic arteries, a risk of blood clots, ear problems, severe osteoporosis, or cervical spondylitis should avoid some inverted poses.

Although yoga during pregnancy is safe if practiced under expert guidance, pregnant women should avoid certain poses that may be problematic.

Training, Licensing, and Certification

There are many training programs for yoga teachers throughout the country. These programs range from a few days to more than 2 years. Standards for teacher training and certification differ depending on the style of yoga.

There are organizations that register yoga teachers and training programs that have complied with minimum educational standards. For example, one nonprofit group requires at least 200 hours of training, with a specified number of hours in areas including techniques, teaching methodology, anatomy, physiology, and philosophy. However, there are currently no official or well-accepted licensing requirements for yoga teachers in the United States.

If You Are Thinking About Yoga

Do not use yoga as a replacement for conventional care or to postpone seeing a doctor about a medical problem.

If you have a medical condition, consult with your health care provider before starting yoga.

Ask about the physical demands of the type of yoga in which you are interested, as well as the training and experience of the yoga teacher you are considering.

Look for published research studies on yoga for the health condition you are interested in.

Tell your health care providers about any complementary and alternative practices you use. Give them a full picture of what you do to manage your health. This will help ensure coordinated and safe care.

NCCAM-Funded Research

Recent studies supported by NCCAM have been investigating yoga's effects on:

Women in yoga class

Courtesy of National Institute on Aging

Blood pressure

Chronic low-back pain

Chronic obstructive pulmonary disease

Depression

Diabetes risk

HIV

Immune function

Inflammatory arthritis and knee osteoarthritis

Insomnia

Multiple sclerosis

Smoking cessation.

Relieving asthma symptoms.

Appendix A: Internet Resources / Further Reading

The following Internet resources may be helpful in answering any health or medical questions you may have. The sites were chosen because of their superior content, accuracy, and authority

CVS Support.

Cyclic Vomiting Syndrome Association
http://www.cvsaonline.org/

Print Publications Online

American Family Physician

http://www.aafp.org/online/en/home/publications/journals/afp.html
A full-text, online version of the esteemed journal. Contains excellent review articles on clinical medicine. Many come with patient education information.

Merck Manual of Diagnosis and Therapy, 17th ed.

http://www.merck.com/mmpe/index.html

A medical guide for professionals, available online. Contains technical information for a host of diseases along with their corresponding diagnosis and treatment suggestions.

Merck Manual of Geriatrics

http://www.merck.com/mkgr/mmg/home.jsp

Similar in format to the Merck Manual of Diagnosis and Therapy, this guide focuses on disorders and diseases with a slant towards implications for the elderly.

Merck Manual of Medical Information - 2nd Home Edition

http://www.merck.com/mmhe/index.html

A consumers' guide to diseases and their treatments. This is a complete online version of the text edition, with videos and a pronunciation guide

Postgraduate Medicine

http://www.postgradmed.com/
Professional medical journal with review articles on diseases and treatments. Although this is directed to the professional, the journal includes patient notes which are directed toward the general consumer.

MEDLINE/MedlinePlus

http://www.nlm.nih.gov/medlineplus/

Anatomy videos aimed at the general consumer plus thousands of articles on a variety of health related topics.

PubMed

http://www.ncbi.nlm.nih.gov/sites/entrez
PubMed comprises more than 20 million citations for biomedical literature from MEDLINE, life science journals, and online books. Citations may include links to full-text content from PubMed Central and publisher web sites.

News Services

These sources offer reliable information and up to date news stories about medical research.

Understanding Medical News

Consumer's Guide to Taking Charge of Medical Information

http://www.health-insight-harvard.org/

This guide, developed by the Harvard School of Public Health, helps you to decipher "scary" headlines.

Deciphering Medspeak

http://mlanet.org/resources/medspeak/index.html

To make informed health decisions, you have probably read a newspaper or magazine article, tuned into a radio or television program, or searched the Internet to find answers to health questions. If so, you have probably encountered "medspeak," the specialized language of health professionals. The Medical Library Association developed "Deciphering Medspeak" to help translate common "medspeak" terms.

HealthNewsReviews

http://www.healthnewsreview.org/
HealthNewsReview.org is a website dedicated to: Improving the accuracy of news stories about medical treatments, tests, products and procedures.

Helping consumers evaluate the evidence for and against new ideas in health care.

Interpreting News on Diet and Nutrition

http://www.hsph.harvard.edu/nutritionsource/nutrition-news/media/

Confused by all the conflicting stories about what's good to eat and what's not? Sensational headlines don't always tell the whole story. Look at how nutrition news fits into the bigger scientific picture.

·

Understanding Risk. What Do Those Headlines Really Mean?

http://www.niapublications.org/tipsheets/pdf/Understanding_Risk-What_Do_Those_Headlines_Really_Mean.pdf

Tipsheet that discusses the differences among types of clinical research and explains the significance of types of risk in research results. Excellent easy to understand information about risk.

Beyond the Headlines: What Consumers Need To Know About Nutrition News

http://www.foodinsight.org/

The International Food Information Council Foundation is dedicated to the mission of effectively communicating science-based information on health, food safety and nutrition for the public good.

Recommended Online News Sources

Aetna InteliHealth Health News

http://www.intelihealth.com/IH/ihtIH/WSIHW000/333/333.html?k=menux408x333

Top news headlines for the day. There is a section with commentaries written by Harvard Medical School physicians of several of the day's top news stories.

CNN Health

http://www.cnn.com/HEALTH/

Daily updated articles from a variety of news sources with links to related CNN stories and websites.

1st Headlines - Top Health Headlines

http://www.1stheadlines.com/health.htm

Top news stories from a variety of sources. Story may be covered by more than one news sources, allowing you to compare stories and fill in information gaps.

Reuters Health eLine

http://www.reutershealth.com/en/index.html

Daily medical news for the consumer (free) and for the professional (requires a subscription fee).

News Sources with Daily or Weekly Email Delivery

MedlinePlus Health News

http://www.nlm.nih.gov/medlineplus/

Produced by the National Library of Medicine, this site has daily news releases from sources such as United Press International, New York Times Syndicate, and Reuters. Stories can be retrieved for thirty days from publication. Users may sign up for daily email of "Health Headlines" in several different categories.

Medscape

http://www.medscape.com/

From WebMD, a website for doctors with a comprehensive news feature. Go to the website to read the daily news or sign up for any of the forty free newsletters for delivery to your email address. There are newsletters in twenty-five specialties, a weekly multi-specialty edition, health business news, and much more.

NewsWise

http://feeds.feedburner.com/NewswiseMednews
Medical news stories. Information from news releases of more than four hundred universities, professional associations, and research institutions. Register and sign up to receive weekly medical news digests via email.

Alternative Medicine Ask Dr. Weil

http://www.drweil.com/

The popular doctor discusses alternative healing remedies for many common ailments.

Alternative Medicine Homepage

http://www.pitt.edu/~cbw/altm.html
From the Falk Library of the Health Sciences, University of Pittsburgh - a jumpstation for sources of information on unconventional, alternative, complementary, innovative, and integrative therapies.

HerbMed

http://www.herbmed.org/

HerbMed is an interactive, electronic herbal database. It provides hyperlinked access to the scientific & medical research articles on the use of herbs for treating medical conditions. This evidence-based information resource is for
professionals, researchers, and the general public.

National Center for Complementary and Alternative Medicine

http://nccam.nih.gov/

General information about alternative and complementary therapies with links to research studies currently being conducted on alternative therapies for a variety of conditions.

Rosenthal Center for Complementary and Alternative Medicine

http://www.rosenthal.hs.columbia.edu//

Links to resources on acupuncture, homeopathy, chiropractic, and herbal medicine and alternative therapies for cancer and women's health. The Center sponsors research on alternative and complementary medical practices.

Clinical Research Trials

Center Watch

http://www.centerwatch.com/

Information on over 41,000 clinical trials for twenty disease categories. Profiles of 150 research centers conducting clinical trials and profiles of companies that provide a variety of contract services to the clinical trials industry. Includes industry and government sponsored clinical trials and information on new drug treatments approved by the Food and Drug Administration.

Clinical Trials

http://www.clinicaltrials.gov/

Information on current research being conducted on treatments for different diseases. Browse by disease category and sponsor or search the entire site. Learn what clinical trials are all about and how to decide to participate in a trial.

Diseases, Medical Conditions, General Health

Aetna Intelihealth

http://www.intellihealth.com/IH/ihtIH?t=408

From the Harvard Medical School, information on diseases and medical conditions, health and fitness, medications, nutrition, childbirth, and other topics.

Healthfinder

http://www.healthfinder.gov/

From the U.S. Department of Health and Human Services, a gateway to consumer information on diseases, medical conditions, health promotion, and many other topics.

Mayo Clinic

http://www.mayoclinic.com/

From the famed Mayo Clinic, information on diseases and conditions, treatment decisions, drugs and supplements, healthy living, and health assessment tools. Special features include online videos of exercises, diagnostic tests, surgical procedures, and medical conditions, healthy recipes, and self-care information.

National Organization for Rare Diseases

http://www.rarediseases.org/

Basic information on rare diseases and disorders. Full-reports are available for a fee.

NOAH (New York Online Access to Health)
http://www.noah-health.org/
English and Spanish language information and resources from organizations and governmental agencies. Aging, cancer, asthma, eye diseases, foot and ankle disorders, and pain are just a few of the topics covered.

Health Care Providers

American Board of Medical Specialties (ABMS)
http://www.abms.org/

Verify the certification status of any physician in the 24 specialities of the ABMS. Registration is required (free) and user is limited to five searches in a 24 hour period.

AMA Physician Select
https://extapps.ama-assn.org/doctorfinder/recaptcha.jsp

Gives credentials of MD's and DO's including medical school, year of graduation, and specialties.

American Hospital Directory

http://www.ahd.com/
Profiles of U.S. hospitals. Basic service is free; more detailed information by paid subscription only.

Federation of State Medical Boards

http://www.fsmb.org/

Select "Public Services" from the left-hand index, then select "Directory of State Medical Boards" to find links to web sites for the 50 U.S. States, plus the District of Columbia, Guam, and the Northern Mariana Islands. Not all of the states have physician profile or disciplinary action information. There are also links to osteopathic physician sites when available.

Health Pages

http://www.healthpages.com/

Information about physicians, dentists, hospitals and clinics, elder care facilities, dietitians and nutritionists.

Joint Commission on the Accreditation of Healthcare Organizations

http://www.jointcommission.org/
The Quality Check feature on this site supplies details on individual hospital performance ratings from JCAHO's accreditation reports. View Performance

Reports and compare institutions' ratings. Reports cover hospitals, nursing homes, ambulatory care facilities, home care, laboratory services, and long term care facilities.

Nursing Home Compare

http://www.medicare.gov/NHCompare/Include/DataSection/Questions/SearchCriteriaNEW.asp?version=default&browser=Chrome|6|WinNT&language=English&defaultstatus=0&pagelist=Home&CookiesEnabledStatus=True

Provides detailed information about the performance of every Medicare and Medicaid certified nursing home in the country. Searchable by state. Includes a guide to choosing a nursing home and a nursing home checklist to help in making informed choices.

Questions and Answers about Health Insurance: A Consumer Guide

http://www.ahrq.gov/consumer/insuranceqa/

Questions and answers on choosing and using a health plan.

Quackery and Health Fraud

Quackwatch

http://www.quackwatch.com/

Want information about whether those alternative therapies work? This site has information on health fraud, medical quackery, "new age" medicine and "alternative" and "complementary" medicine.

National Council against Health Fraud

http://www.ncahf.org/
Non-profit voluntary health agency focusing on health fraud, misinformation, and quackery as public health oncerns. Read their position papers on acupuncture, homepathy, chiropractic, and other health issues.

Surgery

American College of Surgeons

http://www.facs.org/
   Public information section offers guidelines on choosing a qualified surgeon.

Tests and Procedures - MedlinePlus

http://www.nlm.nih.gov/medlineplus/tutorial.html
Interactive tutorials on 24 common tests and diagnostic procedures and more than 30 surgeries and treatment procedures.

Glossary of Medical Terms

Abnormal: Not normal. Deviating from the usual position, condition, structure or behavior. An abnormal growth could indicate a premalignant or malignant condition. In other words, an abnormal growth could indicate cancer

Acquired: An acquired condition is one that isn't present at birth. In other words, it is a condition that is not inherited.

Acute: A condition with an abrupt onset. A brain aneurism is said to be acute if it comes on suddenly. An acute condition could also describe an illness of short duration that rapidly progresses and requires urgent care.

Airway: The trachea. A method of preventing sensation, used to eliminate pain. The loss or prevention of pain, as caused by anesthesia.

Aneurysm or Aneurism: An abnormal blood-filled swelling of an artery or vein, resulting from a localized weakness in the wall of the vessel.

Angiography: A medical imaging technique in which an X-ray image is taken to visualize the inside of blood vessels and organs of the body, with particular interest in the arteries, veins and the heart chambers.

Artery: An efferent blood vessel from the heart, conveying blood away from the heart regardless of oxygenation status.

Autopsy: A dissection performed on a cadaver to find possible cause(s) of death. An after-the-fact examination, especially of the causes of a failure.

Berry aneurysm: An aneurism that looks like a berry. It usually happens where a cerebral artery leaves the circular artery at the base of the brain.

Blood pressure: The pressure exerted by the blood against the walls of the arteries and veins; it varies during the heartbeat cycle, and according to a person's age, health and physical condition. The great majority of people who have serious conditions from high blood pressure suffer debilitating illness.

Brain: The control center of the central nervous system of an animal located in the skull which is responsible for perception, cognition, attention, memory, emotion, and action.

Brain aneurysm: See berry aneurysm.

Brain swelling: See: Cerebral edema.

Breathing: The act of respiration; a single instance of this.

Calcium: A mineral stored in the bones. Calcium is added to bones by osteoblasts and is removed osteoclasts. This mineral s essential for healthy bones and regulates muscle contraction, heart action, nervous system maintenance, and normal blood clotting. Food sources of calcium include dairy foods, some leafy green vegetables such as broccoli and collards, canned salmon, clams, oysters, calcium-fortified foods, and tofu.

Calcium channel blocker: A drug that blocks calcium from entering the heart and artery muscle, preventing narrowing of the arteries.

Cardiovascular: Relating to the circulatory system, that is the heart and blood vessels.

Catheter: small tube inserted into a body cavity to remove fluid, create an opening, distend a passageway or administer a drug

Cell: The basic unit of a living organism, surrounded by a cell membrane.

Cerebral: Of, or relating to the brain or cerebral cortex of the brain.

Cerebral aneurysm: See: Berry aneurysm.

Cholesterol: A sterollipid synthesized by the liver and transported in the bloodstream to the membranes of all animal cells; it plays a central role in many biochemical processes and, as a lipoprotein that coats the walls of blood vessels, is associated with cardiovascular disease.

Circle of Willis: An arterial circle at the base of the brain. Circulation: The movement of the blood in the blood-vascular system, by which it is brought into close relations with almost every living elementary constituent.

Cocaine: A stimulant narcotic in the form of a white powder that users generally self-administer by insufflation through the nose. Any derivative of cocaine. Extracted from the leaves of the coca scrub (Erythroxylon coca) indigenous to the Andean highlands of South America.

Coma: A state of sleep from which one may not wake up, usually induced by some form of trauma.

Compression (medicine): Pressing together. As in a compression fracture, nerve compression, or spinal cord compression.

Compression (embryology): To shorten in time.

Connective tissue: type of tissue found in animals whose main function is binding other tissue systems (such as muscle to skin) or organs and consists of the following three elements: cells, fibers and a ground substance (or extracellular matrix).

Contrast: Any substance, such as barium sulfate, used in radiography to increase the visibility of internal structures

CT scan: Computerized tomography scan. Pictures of the body created by a computer where multiple X-ray images are turned into pictures on a screen.

Cysts: A pouch or sac without opening, usually membranous and containing morbid matter, which develops in one of the natural cavities or in the substance of an organ.

Dizziness: he state of being dizzy; the sensation of instability.

Doppler ultrasound: A type of ultrasound that detects and measures blood flow.

Ehlers-Danlos syndrome: A heritable disorder of connective tissue with easy bruising, joint hypermobility (loose joints), skin laxity, and weakness of tissues.

Emergency department: The department of a hospital that treats emergencies.

Extended family: a family consisting of parents and children, along with either grandparents, grandchildren, aunts or uncles etc.

Extremity: the most extreme or furthest point of something.

An extreme measure.   1.

A hand or foot.   2.

Genetic: (genetics) relating to genetics or genes. Caused by genes.

Groin: The long narrow depression of the human body that separates the trunk from the legs.

Headache: A pain or ache in the head.

Hemorrhage: A heavy release of blood within or from the body.

High blood pressure: Hypertension: a repeatedly elevated blood pressure exceeding 140 over 90 mmHg -- a systolic pressure above 140 with a diastolic pressure above 90.

Inheritance: The hereditary passing of biological attributes from ancestors to their offspring.

Interventional: Intervening, interfering or interceding with the intent of modifying the outcome. For example, an interventional radiologist.

Intracranial: f or pertaining to the brain or inside of the head. Within the cranium.

Kidney: an organ in the body that produces urine.

Lifetime risk: The risk of developing a particular disease or dying from that disease during your lifetime.

Long-term memory: Permanent storage, management, and retrieval of information for later use.

Lumbar: Related to the lower back or loin.

Lumbar puncture: A diagnostic and at times therapeutic procedure performed to collect a sample of cerebrospinal fluid for biochemical, microbiological, and cytological analysis, or rarely to relieve increased intracranial pressure.

Marfan syndrome: A genetic disorder of the connective tissue that causes defects in the heart valves and aorta. Characterized by abnormalities of the eyes, skeleton, and cardiovascular system.

Memory: 1. The ability to recover information about past events or knowledge. 2. The process of recovering information about past events or knowledge. 3. Cognitive reconstruction. The brain engages in a remarkable reshuffling process in an attempt to extract what is general and what is particular about each passing moment.

Migraine: Usually, periodic attacks of headaches on one or both sides of the head. These may be accompanied by nausea, vomiting, increased sensitivity of the eyes to light (photophobia), increased sensitivity to sound (phonophobia), dizziness, blurred vision, cognitive disturbances, and other symptoms. Some migraines do not include headache, and migraines may or may not be preceded by an aura.

MRI: Abbreviation and nickname for magnetic resonance imaging. For more information, see: Magnetic Resonance Imaging; Paul C. Lauterbur ; Peter Mansfield .

Nausea: Nausea, is the urge to vomit. It can be brought by many causes including, systemic illnesses, such as influenza, medications, pain, and inner ear disease. When nausea and/or vomiting are persistent, or when they are accompanied by other severe symptoms such as abdominal pain, jaundice , fever, or bleeding, a physician should be consulted.

Neck: The part of the body joining the head to the shoulders. Also, any narrow or constricted part of a bone or organ that joins its parts as, for example, the neck of the femur bone.

Nerve: A bundle of fibers that uses chemical and electrical signals to transmit sensory and motor information from one body part to another. See: Nervous system.

Nerve cell: See: Neuron.

Neurofibromatosis: A genetic disorder of the nervous system that primarily affects the development and growth of neural (nerve) cell tissues, causes tumors to grow on nerves, and may produce other abnormalities.

Neurological: Having to do with the nerves or the nervous system.

Neurology: The medical specialty concerned with the diagnosis and treatment of disorders of the nervous system -- the brain, the spinal cord, and the nerves.

Neuroradiology: The field within radiology that specializes in the use of radioactive substances, x-rays and scanning devices for the diagnosis and treatment of diseases of the nervous system. Neuroradiology involves the clinical imaging, therapy, and basic science of the central and peripheral nervous system , including but not limited to the brain, spine , head and neck , interventional procedures, techniques in imaging and intervention , and related educational, socioeconomic, and medicolegal issues.

Neurosurgeon: A physician trained in surgery of the nervous system and who specializes in surgery on the brain and other parts of the nervous system. Sometimes called a "brain surgeon."

NIH: The National Institutes of Health. The NIH is an important U.S. health agency. It is devoted to medical research. Administratively under the Department of Health and Human Services (HHS), the NIH consists of 20-some separate Institutes and Centers. NIH's program activities are represented by these Institutes and Centers.

Onset: In medicine, the first appearance of the signs or symptoms of an illness as, for example, the onset of rheumatoid arthritis. There is always an onset to a disease but never to the return to good health. The default setting is good health.

Outpatient: A patient who is not an inpatient (not hospitalized) but instead is cared for elsewhere -- as in a doctor's office, clinic, or day surgery center. The term outpatient dates back at least to 1715. Outpatient care today is also called ambulatory care.

Pain: An unpleasant sensation that can range from mild, localized discomfort to agony. Pain has both physical and emotional components. The physical part of pain results from nerve stimulation. Pain may be contained to a discrete area, as in an injury, or it can be more diffuse, as in disorders like fibromyalgia. Pain is mediated by specific nerve fibers that carry the pain impulses to the brain where their conscious appreciation may be modified by many factors.

Pharmacy: A location where prescription drugs are sold. A pharmacy is, by law, constantly supervised by a licensed pharmacist.

Polycystic kidney disease: One of the genetic disorders characterized by the development of innumerable cysts in the kidneys. These cysts are filled with fluid, and replace much of the mass of the kidneys. This reduces kidney function, leading to kidney failure.

Pupil: The opening of the iris. The pupil may appear to open (dilate) and close (constrict) but it is really the iris that is the prime mover; the pupil is merely the absence of iris. The pupil determines how much light is let into the eye. Both pupils are usually of equal size. If they are not, that is termed anisocoria (from "a-", not + "iso", equal + "kore", pupil = not equal pupils).

Radiologic: Having to do with radiology.

Radiologist: A physician specialized in radiology, the branch of medicine that uses ionizing and nonionizing radiation for the diagnosis and treatment of disease.

Residual: Something left behind. With residual disease, the disease has not been eradicated.

Risk factor: Something that increases a person's chances of developing a disease.

Rupture: A break or tear in any organ (such as the spleen) or soft tissue (such as the achilles tendon). Rupture of the appendix is more likely among uninsured and minority children when they develop appendicitis.

Saccular: From the Latin "sacculus" meaning a small pouch. As for example the alveolar saccules (little air pouches) within the lungs.

Saccular aneurysm: An aneurysm that resembles a small sack. A berry aneurysm is typically saccular. An aneurysm is a localized widening (dilatation) of an artery, vein, or the heart. At the area of an aneurysm, there is typically a bulge and the wall is weakened and may rupture. The word "aneurysm" comes from the Greek "aneurysma" meaning "a widening."

Scan: As a noun, the data or image obtained from the examination of organs or regions of the body by gathering information with a sensing device.

Seizure: Uncontrolled electrical activity in the brain, which may produce a physical convulsion, minor physical signs, thought disturbances, or a combination of symptoms.

Sensitivity: 1. In psychology, the quality of being sensitive. As, for example, sensitivity training, training in small groups to develop a sensitive awareness and understanding of oneself and of ones relationships with others. 2. In disease epidemiology, the ability of a system to detect epidemics and other changes in disease occurrence. 3. In screening for a disease, the proportion of persons with the disease who are correctly identified by a screening test. 4. In the definition of a disease, the proportion of persons with the disease who are correctly identified by defined criteria.

Skull: The skull is a collection of bones which encase the brain and give form to the head and face. The bones of the skull include the following: the frontal, parietal, occipital, temporal, sphenoid, ethmoid, zygomatic, maxilla, nasal, vomer, palatine, inferior concha, and mandible.

Spasm: A brief, automatic jerking movement. A muscle spasm can be quite painful, with the muscle clenching tightly. A spasm of the coronary artery can cause angina. Spasms in various types of tissue may be caused by stress, medication, over-exercise, or other factors.

Spinal cord: The major column of nerve tissue that is connected to the brain and lies within the vertebral canal and from which the spinal nerves emerge. Thirty-one pairs of spinal nerves originate in the spinal cord: 8 cervical, 12 thoracic , 5 lumbar, 5 sacral, and 1 coccygeal. The spinal cord and the brain constitute the central nervous system (CNS). The spinal cord consists of nerve fibers that transmit impulses to and from the brain. Like the brain, the spinal cord is covered by three connective-tissue envelopes called the meninges . The space between the outer and middle envelopes is filled with cerebrospinal fluid (CSF), a clear colorless fluid that cushions the spinal cord against jarring shock. Also known simply as the cord.

Spinal tap: Also known as a lumbar puncture or "LP", a spinal tap is a procedure whereby spinal fluid is removed from the spinal canal for the purpose of diagnostic testing. It is particularly helpful in the diagnosis of inflammatory diseases of the central nervous system, especially infections, such as meningitis. It can also provide clues to the diagnosis of stroke, spinal cord tumor and cancer in the central nervous system.

Stress: Forces from the outside world impinging on the individual. Stress is a normal part of life that can help us learn and grow. Conversely, stress can cause us significant problems.

Stroke: The sudden death of some brain cells due to a lack of oxygen when the blood flow to the brain is impaired by blockage or rupture of an artery to the brain. A stroke is also called a cerebrovascular accident or, for short, a CVA.

Subarachnoid: Literally, beneath the arachnoid, the middle of three membranes that cover the central nervous system. In practice, subarachnoid usually refers to the space between the arachnoid and the pia mater, the innermost membrane surrounding the central nervous system.

Subarachnoid hemorrhage: Bleeding within the head into the space between two membranes that surround the brain. The bleeding is beneath the arachnoid membrane and just above the pia mater. (The arachnoid is the middle of three membranes around the brain while the pia mater is the innermost one.)

Surgery: The word "surgery" has multiple meanings. It is the branch of medicine concerned with diseases and conditions which require or are amenable to operative procedures. Surgery is the work done by a surgeon. By analogy, the work of an editor wielding his pen as a scalpel is s form of surgery. A surgery in England (and some other countries) is a physician's or dentist's office.

Swelling of the brain: See: Cerebral edema.

Symptom: Any subjective evidence of disease. Anxiety, lower back pain, and fatigue are all symptoms. They are sensations only the patient can perceive. In contrast, a sign is objective evidence of disease. A bloody nose is a sign. It is evident to the patient, doctor, nurse and other observers.

Syndrome: A set of signs and symptoms that tend to occur together and which reflect the presence of a particular disease or an increased chance of developing a particular disease.

Temple: An area just behind and to the side of the forehead and the eye, above the side of the check bone (the zygomatic arch) and in front of the ear.

Tension: 1) The pressure within a vessel, such as blood pressure: the pressure within the blood vessels. For example, elevated blood pressure is referred to as hypertension. 2) Stress, especially stress that is translated into clenched scalp muscles and bottled-up emotions or anxiety. This is the type of tension blamed for tension headaches.

Therapeutic: Relating to therapeutics, that part of medicine concerned specifically with the treatment of disease. The therapeutic dose of a drug is the amount needed to treat a disease.

Throat: The throat is the anterior (front) portion of the neck beginning at the back of the mouth , consisting anatomically of the pharynx and larynx . The throat contains the trachea and a portion of the esophagus.

Tobacco: A South American herb, formally known as Nicotiana tabacum, whose leaves contain 2-8% nicotine and serve as the source of smoking and smokeless tobacco.

Transcranial: Through the cranium. As, for example, in transcranial magnetic stimulation.

Ultrasound : High-frequency sound waves. Ultrasound waves can be bounced off of tissues using special devices. The echoes are then converted into a picture called a sonogram. Ultrasound imaging, referred to as ultrasonography, allows physicians and patients to get an inside view of soft tissues and body cavities, without using invasive techniques. Ultrasound is often used to examine a fetus during pregnancy There is no convincing evidence for any danger from ultrasound during pregnancy.

Vessel: A tube in the body that carries fluids: blood vessels or lymph vessels.

Visual field: The entire area that can be seen when the eye is directed forward, including that which is seen with peripheral vision.

X-ray: 1. High-energy radiation with waves shorter than those of visible light. X-rays possess the properties of penetrating most substances (to varying extents), of acting on a photographic film or plate (permitting radiography), and of causing a fluorescent screen to give off light (permitting fluoroscopy). In low doses X-rays are used for making images that help to diagnose disease, and in high doses to treat cancer. Formerly called a Roentgen ray. 2. An image obtained by means of X-rays.

References

1. ^ "Gastroscopy - examination of oesophagus and stomach by endoscope". BUPA. December 2006. Retrieved 2007-10-07.
2. ^ National Digestive Diseases Information Clearinghouse (November 2004). "Upper Endoscopy". National Institutes of Health. Retrieved 2007-10-07.
3. ^ "What is Upper GI Endoscopy?". Patient Center -- Procedures. American Gastroenterological Association. Archived from the original on 2007-09-28. Retrieved 2007-10-07.
4. Wikipedia: http://en.wikipedia.org/wiki/Small_bowel_follow-through
5. Wikipedia: http://en.wikipedia.org/wiki/Upper_GI_series
6. Wikipedia: http://en.wikipedia.org/wiki/Abdominal_ultrasonography
1. ^ Bisset (1 January 2008). Differential Diagnosis in Abdominal Ultrasound, 3/e. Elsevier India. pp. 257. ISBN 9788131215746. Retrieved 10 April 2011.

Printed in Great Britain
by Amazon